I0441339

The Real
Puberty to Sunset

by Thelma Wright

The Real / Puberty to Sunset
Copyright © 2009 by Thelma Wright. All rights reserved.

This title is also available as a Thelma Wright product. Visit www.thelmawright.com for more information.

No part of this publication may be reproduced, stored in a retrieval system to be transmitted in any way by any means, electronic, mechanical, photocopy, recording or otherwise without the prior permission of the author except as provide by USA copyright law.

Scripture quotations are taken from the Holy Bible, King James Version, Cambridge, 1769. All right reserved.

Edited by JoAnn Tucker
Edited by Anthony Wright

Book design copyright © 2009 by Personal Legends Films, Inc. All rights reserved.

Cover design and interior design by Anthony Wright

Published in the United States of America

ISBN   9781451509656

1. Health: Mind & Body
2. Parenting & Families

Preface

After completing a discussion on my book, *Perfect Health? Combating the fear of Prostate Cancer,* I was approached by a lady who asked me if I could come back and do something for the ladies. As treatment and prevention for most cancers are similar, I think that my new book will reach more people. All of the topics in this book are based on discussions that I've had, in the past two years, with people who were going through these issues. If you look at the table of contents, you will note the various issues that were discussed. Each of these topics, if not handled correctly, can lead to stress and worry. The combination of stress and worry can lead to many medical problems, including cancer. My hope, as I alert the reader of these issues, is that, when confronted with any of these issues, he or she will seek a way of handling them that will lead to less stress.

Table of Contents

Part V: Maturity

Part VI: Lack of Love

Part VII: Death

Part VIII: Challenges

Part IX: Sunset

Dedication

In memory of my mother, Virginia Bryan, who laid the foundation for this book.

Thank You from Author

My first book *Perfect Health? Combating the Fear of Prostate Cancer* has brought me such joy from readers like:

Lavern, R.N., from Georgia who classified it as a great book; much different than others on the subject.

Every one of you that told me that, once you started to read it, you could not put it down.

The unnamed characters, from my book, who called me the minute you got to the page that described you.

To those who cannot wait to read my second book.

Most of all, I would like to give thanks to the people whose lives it has touched in a special way.

To all of you, I say thank you for allowing me to share the perils and prevention of this deadly disease. Please join me in thanking God for His Insight and Guidance as I wrote my story, and I look forward to your continued support as you introduce my books to your family and friends.

Message from Author to Parents

As a society, we are deeply concerned with the negative paths some of our youth are embracing. Our values have changed so much in 40 years. When I was growing up, a teenage girl's primary concerns were achieving her goals and not be blindsided by pregnancy. Many children were brought up in church where morals and good manners were instilled. Being rude to your parents was not tolerated, and parents took parenting seriously. Parents were often classified as strict, caring, or occasionally lacking in parental skills. Never were parents classified by their child as being a "best friend." Most homes had a father present, and for those that did not, an uncle, grandfather or some other older male assumed the role of a father figure. If you dared to be rude to your mother, and she felt you were not taking heed to her discipline, she allowed the surrogate father to enforce the discipline. In many cases, it was not physical; a manly talk went a long way. The parents' goal was to bring their children up to be productive members of society. They dared their children to achieve the many opportunities that were unavailable to them in their youth. Children were pleased to know that their accomplishments would bring joy to their parents. Achievement would preserve or elevate the good standing of the family name; therefore, they worked diligently towards becoming a success.

Today, in trying to be a parent and a friend, discipline is often lacking. Too many children are raised in single-family homes, most of which are run by females who were raised in similar households. An absence of a male influence is becoming a disturbing trend. Having lived in a home where my father was always present, followed by a marriage that lasted over 20 years, I am well aware of the negative impact a single family home can have on some children. If single mothers will remember that Jesus Christ is waiting for them to call on Him for His Help and Guidance, He in turn will lead them to His Father (God). The single mother will be amazed at the positive transformation of her household as the drive and grades of her children will surpass those of many kids raised in two parent homes. God has willingly taken up the role that so many earthly fathers have too easily abandoned.

Jesus Christ died for our sins eliminating the need for us to live in sin and dire need. As churches, we must make sure no child in our congregation is brought up without the influence of a male figure. Putting this practice in place will increase the number of children who attend church. If your church does not have enough men to handle the influx, God will send you the increase.

If you are not a member of a church, find such a person for your child, or sign them up in a program such as Big Brothers / Big Sisters that provides this service. If you fail to do so, your children may seek the friendship and love of the wrong type of male; with negative ramifications.

With so much perversion in our society, you have to be careful when you bring a stranger around to be a part of your child's life. Proper screening is essential. *Keep the line of communication open with your child. Also, look for any negative nonverbal communication. Make sure you do not put negative suggestions in your child's head. Too many of us are not good at monitoring and discussing the non-verbal communication of our children, and children often do not volunteer this information willingly.*

Although unplanned pregnancy is still a major problem for

our youth, they are now faced with many more serious problems that may derail their dreams. Today, many children have no idea what goes on inside a church, and among those that are active members in church, their words or deeds often do not reflect those of someone who knows or follows the scriptures. Some parents have allowed their children to make their own decisions about attending church, and many have decided that church is not for them.

Church influences children to be law-abiding citizens as many of our laws were taken straight from the Holy Bible. This is a surprise to some children. What about His command in *Proverbs 22:6; "**Train up a child in the way he should go; and when he is old he will not depart from it?**"* Yes, some children that were brought up in church do go astray as the prodigal son did, but believe His word, they will return and embrace His teachings again.

With having to work multiple jobs to maintain our lifestyles or survive, too many of our children are raised without adequate supervision. In this vacuum, correct morals are not being taught or enforced. We have rewritten the laws of discipline, ignoring many areas where discipline should be enforced, and later regretting our failure to do so.

As our children enter their teen years, they should be warned that many addictive seductions await them. You should encourage them to use wisdom in choosing their friends. In your effort to be a good parent, you should be aware, that even though you do your best to teach your children to be productive members of society, peer pressure could undermine all your good work. Knowing this, see to it that your teenager spends adequate time with the family, and limit the amount of time they spend with their peers who may easily replace you as their role model.

Many parents will tell you that they were caught off guard when they found out that their son or daughter was addicted to some drug or other vice. As we search our hearts to see how this could have happened, many times we find out that our children have cut class in school without our knowledge. Our work schedule may not allow us to be at home to receive the phone calls from the school reporting their absence.

Have you ever wondered why only the best high school students get to be on the football, basketball, hockey, baseball or other sport team? Of course, there must be a team for the best students, but does that mean that we must forsake the rest? With the great rewards that the best can obtain by making the team, it is no surprise to see many kids go astray if they realize they will not be selected. As parents, when this occurs, we must take pleasure in encouraging them to concentrate on their grades. Maintaining good grades should always be their *goal but* our children are often upset by this disappointment.

Teens can be very cruel towards one another. Many times they give children that are smarter or different a hard time, and the offended often suffer in silence. As parents, even though we know this goes on in schools, we seldom question our children to see if they are experiencing it. I believe, if we teach our children that if they want a friend they have to become one first, they will be able to seek out positive friends who will stand up for them when they are being ridiculed. *Have you inquired about what is going on in your child's classroom lately?* A parent should arrange to visit their child's classroom each term to see how the child acts in school. It will be good for the parent, teacher and child.

I believe that the many hours I have spent in church, in various leadership roles, have helped me to make some positive choices. At times when I stood alone, I knew I was never really alone. When Jesus Christ returned to heaven, He said he will be with us always.

Matthew 28:19-20:
Go ye therefore, and teach all nations, baptizing them in the name of the Father, and the Son, and the Holy Ghost. Teaching them to observe all things whatsoever I have commanded you: and lo I am with you always, even unto the end

of the world.

Recently, I asked some of my friends if they remembered how we became friends. Most of them said I approached them first. I was not aware of this, but I am thankful I did. I have had positive friends throughout all stages of my life.

Try to read a book a couple of times a year with your teen and discuss the contents when completed. Today, many books come in audio form, so that is an alternative that may fit into your busy schedule. This will allow you to be a part of your teenager's life while giving sound parental advice along the way. Until your child is able to be financially responsible for his or her upkeep, find a way of always being a focal part of your child's life; after all, you are the provider of his or her needs. The positive results from your good parental skills will bring you a sense of satisfaction.

Many teens depend totally on their parents for their support but refuse to let their parents know what is going on in their social lives. This is a bad practice. Should something negative happen to the teen, the bewildered parents have no idea who their child hung out with or who to turn to for help.

Time passes swiftly and eventually it will be time for your child to move on to college. As your child approaches this age, discuss your child's plans with him or her. Although some children have no intention of becoming good scholars, they may want to go out of town to some expensive school with you footing the bill. Stand your ground. Insist on a school near home until you see your child is serious about studying.

If you are blessed to raise your children in a Godly home, and they did not stray too far away from your teachings, they will continue to serve God as they enter adulthood. I know you give God blessings for His grace.

Part I
Puberty

The Story

In the hill near our house in Barbados, there were these wild, beautiful, yellow flowers that bloomed a certain time of year. If you took a walk at dawn, it was very beautiful to observe rows of them as they swayed in the wind. After ten o'clock, that same morning, they were all wilted and seemed to be fast asleep, only to open up and sway in the cool breeze in their full beauty the next morning. This continued for a few weeks and then they disappeared. The beauty and dance of those flowers made me think of puberty. Their closure and reopening remind me of the different stages we go through in life, until the final closure. As puberty is usually described as a time when children blossom, as they start the process of becoming men or women, I believe it is only fitting that I start my story beginning at puberty and finish when we no longer bloom.

From Puberty...

Proverbs: 8:17: God says:
"I love them that love me; and those that seek me early
shall find me."

This world consists of good (God) who desires you to serve Him and evil (the Devil) who wants to take control over you; being aware of this, the choice is yours to decide which path you will take.

Growing up can be so much fun. You skip; you jump and even pretend to fly. You often baffle your parents with your inquiries. When asked what you want to be when you grow up, you present at least two or more choices. There is not much that you think about that you will not share with your parents, and your parents hope that this free-flowing communication will continue. Sadly, for many, this is short lived and stops as soon as puberty starts.

You may have heard of the days when some mothers did not prepare their daughters for the onset of their menses, and their daughters thought they were struck with some deadly disease when it commenced. This is not as widespread today, as increased education, coupled with the invention of the disposable sanitary napkins/pads, have made today's girls more prepared to approach their menses.

As a little girl, your body starts to change. Some girls start this process at nine years old or younger. Your breast begins to enlarge and hair begins to grow under your arms and on your pubic area. Soon, you noticed that your vagina begins to get moist with secretions and before long you start to menstruate. This may occur before the subject is taught in your class. If your class discussed menstruation, instead of giggling, you wished you had paid close attention. What did the teacher say? Oh yes, she said, "as a female, I was born with two ovaries that have eggs, and once a month one or more egg ovulates and enters the lining of the uterus. Shedding of this lining and blood, leads to bleeding through the vagina or a period as it is commonly called. This means I will get a monthly period that can last from two to seven days." Now you begin to hope that for you a period will be a normal event. For others it might not be so, as the teacher had stated, it can be a painful and uncomfortable time for some girls. Now is the time for you to see your parent, guardian or school nurse who will teach you how to apply your sanitary napkins. It is important to take daily baths or perform genital care, and change your pads every three to four hours as necessary during your period. Some girls go though this stage without discussing these changes with their parents and turn to an older sister or a friend for advice instead. Now your parents wished that discussing sex and the reproductive system with you would have been easier. They know you are not discussing what is going in your body with them and wonder what they can say or do to gain your trust.

Girls should be taught that their bodies have matured and pregnancy can occur if they have unprotected sex. Many parents introduce their daughters to birth control at this time, but this should not be interpreted as giving permission to indulge in sexual activity. Abstinence should always be encouraged. *Why? It is the right thing to do. Should your child comply, in time, she will thank you for your guidance.*

Now you notice your friends, in or near your age group, are going through similar changes; yet some more pronounced than others. This is around the time where you and your peers start to compare how every one in your class is developing. As teenagers, your bluntness sometimes hurt those who you criticized negatively. This behavior should be discouraged, as it has caused many young girls to undergo cosmetic surgeries, to correct the parts of their bodies they were teased about.

Feeling comfortable in your body is very important. Make sure you eat a balanced nutritious diet that consists of all the following foods: whole grains, vegetables, fruits, meats, beans, milk and oils. Include some plain water as part of your daily drinks; stay away from too many sweets and fried foods; get plenty of exercise and adequate sleep, and do your best to keep your body and mind healthy. Learning to love and take care of your body at an early age may keep you from a lifetime of worry. Remember, before you were born God knew your shape, now it is your turn to look after His gift.

Some of the changes that go on in **a boys' body** at puberty are different than that of a girl's. As a boy, you notice your voice begins to change; the pitch varies in different individuals. Some boys' voices become higher in its pitch, and others, a very deep base. This can occur at the age of twelve or earlier. Many boys, because of teasing, try to speak very little during this phase. Thankfully, for most of you, this only lasts for a short period of time. At this stage, you also start to grow facial and chest hair. Then you wake up one morning and your penis has increased in size almost overnight. Some boys become more endowed than others. If you do not have the opportunity to observe this in your sibling as a normal process, it might appear as something weird, when you wake up one morning with a penile erection. Before long, you may have what some describe as a "wet dream." This is a normal process in which semen produced by the male hormonal glands ejaculates. Semen is a clear white or light grey sticky fluid that passes through the urethra, which is the same tube in the penis that your urine passes through. This signifies you are a young man potentially capable of fathering a child. Embrace these changes, all healthy boys go through them. Good hygiene is very important at this stage, and if you are uncircumcised (meaning the foreskin from your penis was not removed) do not forget to retract your foreskin and wash and dry the area well when you bathe or perform genital care. *Your parents might discuss birth* *control at this stage, but abstinence should be practiced.* **Yes, it is possible**.

Just like your female counterparts, you, too, have been blessed with special genes that were predetermined before you were born. There is and only will be one you. So do your best to look after your body with a well-balanced nutritional diet, plenty of outdoor play, and exercise. Most guys like to be six feet tall or more, and boys usually reach their predetermined height much later than girls. I encourage you to love the new you, even if you do not attain your desired height. Boys, especially those that play sports, should avoid teasing each other about their physical development. Negative comments can remain with the offended for years, and, at times, bring out negative behavior that can be harmful to oneself and others.

What Choices Will You Make?

Joshua 24:15:

"And if it seem evil unto you to serve the Lord, choose you this day whom ye will serve; whether the gods which your fathers served that were on the other side of the flood, or the gods of the Amorites, in whose land ye dwell: but as for me and my house we will serve the Lord."

For most of you, these formative years can very well dictate which path your adult life will lead. Peer pressure is very rampant at this stage. Many of you will participate in weird rituals that you know in your heart are wrong, just to be a member of some group. As you are challenged at this phase, there will be many times when not being part of certain groups will turn out to be an excellent choice.

If there is one gift that comes in handy here, it is the "gift of wisdom." Knowing who is most likely to turn out to be a true friend can save you many moments of anguish later. So choose your friends wisely.

Proverbs 27: 17: states:

"Iron sharpeneth iron so a man sharpeneth the countenance of his friend.

"If you are joining a group, usually you have to conform to their ways rather than the other way around."

One very important choice in growing up is dating. As you ponder when to start dating and how far you will go on a date, I will tell you not to hurry and to take your time as you grow up. I believe this is the best advice any parent can give a teenager. Few teens will take this advice as many eagerly look forward to going to the movies and having those long chats on the telephone and emails with that special boy or girl. As you enjoy fun time together, keeping your dates full of innocent fun is encouraged.

Remember, today we live in a world that can be very dangerous; as far as sex is concerned. Many who have experimented with sex at an early age have become teenaged mothers and father, others have had an abortion, or have given their child up for adoption, and some have ended up with a sexually transmitted disease (STD). One STD, called HIV progresses to AIDS, and has taken many young lives. A series of prescribed antibiotics may not cure most STDs today. As you go through this phase, do not be afraid to say "no," and mean "no," to any sexual advances. Most times a teenage crush is just that. If your first love really loves you, he or she will understand why it is important for you not to be pressured.

It is amazing how for centuries many have fallen for the line that says; "if you have sex with me it shows me that you really love me, "only to find out they have just been added to a list of those who are quick to please. As minority girls in the USA continue to lead in the number of newly acquired sexually transmitted diseases, common sense and safety should be the goal of every youth. This is your life. Do your best to protect it and stay spiritually and physically healthy.

I wish I could tell you that all of your sexual advances will come from a member of the opposite sex close to your age. However, as you mature, you may be propositioned by some that are older than you, some that are family members, and others that are the same sex as you. Being forewarned, you should make sure that you are on your guard and say no to any unwarranted advances. *Many carry the scars of trusting someone who has in-*

vaded their space and violated their trust, resulting in haunting memories that just will not go away. **The book of Proverbs has such wisdom and should be read by all teenagers**. This will show you that the challenges you face have been faced by teens for generations before you. How you bypass or conquer these issues is the key to your achieving a life with very few scars.

Dare to be a Positive Leader

Phillipians 4:13
"I can do all things through Christ which strengtheneth me."

Leaders that dare to be different in a positive way can be hard to find. Look around you and see how you can become a positive trendsetter. Your effort may improve the lives of others; bringing you and the persons whose lives you touched many private feelings of gratitude and happiness.

Doing your best should be your goal. Remember if you believe you can do something, chances are you can do it. Be committed to put in the work to see your dreams fulfilled.

Most people do not achieve their best because others have told them their dreams are impossible to obtain. Sometimes it is best not to share your dreams with too many people. Dreams are easier to be realized this way.

Graduate from every class and decide which path you will take after you graduate from high school. Be aware that even if you are an "A" student, thorns will be placed in your way. Dare to conquer all obstacles to achieve your goal.

Aim to Achieve

We are living in a high technological society where machines now perform many jobs previously done by man. In some fields this has decreased the amount of manpower needed. Keeping focus on your education will keep you on the right track. Of course, you should still have lots of fun at this stage. Look for activities that allow you to explore different cultural events that you can enjoy with your family and friends.

Take note of the encouragement of teachers and friends. Many times they can spot your special talent and can give you encouragement that may lead you into a career that can be both rewarding and prosperous. Yes, you may not like their advice but when it becomes a reality, remember to thank them.

Avoid seemingly minor traps that often turn into major setbacks.

Being part of a peer group can sometimes lead to indulging in negative behavior. You might get involved with bullying others or cutting classes. This can lead into doing some illegal activities such as using **drugs** or joining **a gang. Do not allow your dreams to be derailed because of these actions.**

Proverbs 25: 28:
"He that have no rule over his spirit is like a city that is broken down, **and without walls."**

As you look around you, you will see many living examples of those who did not use wisdom to control their actions, they have succumbed to participating in destructive behaviors, which lead to the abuse of alcoholic beverages, smoking, doing drugs, gambling, pornography, prostitution and other behavior that make you loose your true self. Avoid dares to sample any illegal vice to show you are strong enough not to get trapped. Traveling down these addictive paths have robbed many of productive years and may lead to early death. See the following words of Proverbs that forewarns you of overindulgence:

Proverbs 20: 1:
"Wine is a mocker, strong drink is raging and whosoever is deceived thereby is not wise."

Proverbs 23:31-32:
"Look not thou upon wine when it is red, when it giveth his color in the cup, when it moveth itself aright. At the last it biteth like a serpent and stingeth like an adder."

Sadly, many accept negative challenges, and become slaves to these vices. Few can afford the cost of long-term medical and psychological treatment, which can be exorbitant, with no guarantee of a complete recovery. **Some seek solace in the Word of God and believe in Jesus Christ to set them free of their addictions. I find those that are delivered through Jesus Christ stay addiction free longer if they stay in the Word of God.**

Which Path Will You Take for A Higher Education?

Proverbs 3:6
"In all thy ways acknowledge Him (God), and he shall direct thy paths."

That was my father's favorite scripture verse to recite to me. Whenever I was pondering which path to take and I wrote my dad, asking for his opinion, as I eagerly opened his letters the advice never changed. He always directed me to my Source.

Deciding which path to take after you graduate from high school should be decided on before you enter college. This will easily save you time and thousand of dollars in tuition fees. Be aware that if you go to college and have not chosen a career path, you can end up taking many courses that might not be useful in your eventual career choice.

Much thought should be given to your choice of a college or trade school; keeping in mind that tuition is expensive. You should consider this and seek advice on ways to achieve a good education while keeping your cost manageable, if at all possible. Remember, many end up with a good education but have loans that take many years to repay. This can cause stress, which makes enjoying life's pleasures difficult. You may be encouraged to attend a two to four year college or university, *but do not forget about trade schools.* Many offer training that allows you to get into the job market much sooner. Check those offered by your state technical institute first. The *cost can be lower, and placement after graduation may be easier.* Be aware that demand for entry is oftentimes greater than the allotted space. After graduating from these schools, many continue to further their education at a college or university while working in their chosen fields. I do find that those who choose trade schools wisely achieve higher incomes sooner, work with companies that have better benefits, and are prone to start their own business.

How Much Shall You Play in College?

Matthew 10:16
Jesus said; "Behold I send you forth as sheep in the midst of wolves: be ye therefore wise as serpents, and harmless as doves."

At this stage many move far away from home. Higher education is usually their goal; but many distractions come into play. *"So much freedom and mom and dad are no way in sight to put a curfew in place."* It can be so easy to forget why you left home in the first place.

Being handsome, attractive, funny or downright gorgeous, you are forewarned you may lose track of why you are in college. Many end up overindulging in partying, sex, alcohol or drugs. These can sidetrack or abort your efforts to achieve a higher education. If you are a Christian away from church and family, keeping your Christian values can be done. I pray God gives you the strength to do so for *"greater is He that is within you than he that is within the world."*

Always be aware of your surroundings, and find a buddy to accompany you to and from classes. It may be good to team up with more than one person, just in case someone cannot make it to class. As a teenage girl, if a male approaches you in a car, you should resist the temptation to approach the car, and always deny a free ride. Too many girls disappear or are harmed by letting their guard down by approaching or getting into a car driven by a male who seemed harmless.

There is nothing wrong with you if you see many of your pals getting a date soon after they arrived on campus, although, so far, no one has asked you out. If you make completing your education your main priority there will be plenty of time to date. *Have your first date in a public place surrounded by many people. Until you feel safe with your date, this sort of setting will be an appropriate place to meet, as it can protect you from date rape and being enticed to have sexual intercourse before you are ready.*

You should let your date know your expectation before you date. Make sure he or she understands your values and abides by them. If anyone tries to invade your space without your consent, or displays traits you do not want in a date, it will be wise, not to go on a date with that person again.

Part II
Youth

Time Flies

When you entered college it seemed like your degree would take you forever to accomplish. Yet time has passed so quickly; you are graduating with some major goals you want to accomplish.

For some, marriage is number one on your list. You cannot wait to marry your sweetheart who has supported you throughout your studies. You have not given much thought to your school loans, some of which your parents have co-signed for you. Somehow, you believe you will be able to combine being a spouse with pursuing your new career. You reassure your parents that you will take care of the loans, having no idea that most jobs do not pay enough to do this today. So plan well, especially if you know not helping to repay your loans will cause financial distress to your parents.

Some of you want to go into the job market immediately, seeking a position that compensates you well for all the studies you have done, and the money you have invested. You might look at the job market with a long time goal in mind. A career must have hours that allow you adequate time, and compensation for your eventual family. Whatever decision you make, being a part of the job market will bring you many challenges; I wish you well.

Some of you, who have difficulty obtaining that first job, may settle for a career or job that does not justify the time and money you spent on your education. Whatever position you take, be the best employee. If your work place has room for advancement, this can help you to be considered when a better paying position becomes available. Your positive attitude will be a plus to clients, and a pleasure to your coworkers.

Keep in mind that today many people will have plenty careers before they retire. Being aware of this, you should keep your ears open to new opportunities; there are many nonconventional opportunities that offer fabulous rewards. But you have to do your homework, checking out all opportunities thoroughly to make sure you are not getting involved in some illegal scheme. Take note, you should be suspicious of potential career opportunities that do not require real work.

For those who want to become entrepreneurs and start out on your own business venture: many times you will face insufficient funding, but press forward nonetheless. Believing in your business and giving it your best effort go a long way towards your success. If you are blessed with family and friends who will support you in your new venture with a good product and hard work, success is obtainable. As commercial rent continues to increase in most cities, starting a business at home, if your city zoning laws allow it will save you plenty. I believe many small businesses fail because of their high overhead cost. If you came from a family of entrepreneurs, you might consider using your education to help the business to expand, thereby increasing the possibility of having a business that will span many generations. *This is often overlooked, as many prefer to follow their own dreams, only to later realize that helping to build the family business is like a hidden treasure.*

Adult Life

Now you are an adult; monthly bills start to arrive. "What an eye opener!" As soon as you pay your one set of monthly bills, a new set arrives. You begin to wonder how your parents have managed all these years. Many of you graduate from high school or college and you have not been taught how to write a check, balance a checkbook or manage your finances. "How are you going to make sure that you approach your finance in a knowledgeable way?" Getting educated on how to manage your money will save you from many sleepless nights and lots of money problems in the long term. Therefore, those of you who made sure you took a course in finance and know how to apply the knowledge effectively should be one step ahead. For those of you, who have not done this, remember to do so. Seek the advice of a competent person licensed in the area of your needs, and ask them to advice you. Do your homework when seeking such a person. Some depend on word of mouth that such professionals are good without finding out themselves. Make sure the person can discuss how they can help you in language you can understand. Soon it will be time to start to repay your school loans; remember to include these as you set up your budget. What about your parents? Do they manage money wisely or do they live from paycheck to paycheck? If they manage money well, take note and take their advice.

It is amazing how soon your spending habits will change. Instead of buying the most recent designer clothes or sneakers, you will now buy last season's brand. As you begin spending your money instead of your parents, saving becomes very important to you. Knowing how to save money from each paycheck you receive will help you to accomplish your dreams.

If you are working and living at home, do not become a financial burden to your parents. Give a fair monetary contribution towards your upkeep. Too many young adults become financial burdens to their parents while they squander their earnings.

Single Living

Staying single, as you sort out your career is a choice, which will allow you to focus on which path you will take. If used wisely, when you enter into a relationship, this will be a plus. If you must choose a roommate, it is best that the roommate is a friend and not one that you are romantically involved with. Do not play house, that is, do not pretend to be married. Leave that until you are ready. My belief is that anyone who wants a permanent partner on a daily basis needs to get married. You may not agree, but this is God's way.

Time flies as you enjoy climbing your career ladder, you wake up one day and you are ten years older and still single. If you are satisfied with your situation, there is no need to worry. Today, single life is enjoyed by both sexes, so there is a chance when you are ready to settle down you will find a mate.

For African American career women, the choices of a husband can be slim. If you fall into this category, you can widen your horizon by stepping outside of your race; be open to different possibilities. Be assured, men and women have been crossing over for centuries. Yes, you might be concerned about the negative comments and stares of others. You worry that if you have children, they will be ridiculed because of their mixed race. Plus there's the possibility that members from one or both sides of your extended family may not accept your relationship, and may disown you or your children. Remember that although the outer layer of a man's skin comes in different shades, and his hair comes in different textures and colors, man is made the same way internally. This racial discrimination is not new. *Moses crossed over when he married his Ethiopian wife. His brother and sister did not like that he married a woman of color and voiced their opinions.* See:

Numbers 12:1:

"And Miriam and Aaron spoke against Moses because of the Ethiopian woman whom he had married: for he had married an Ethiopian woman."

Moses was comfortable with his choice, and God was angry about the attitude of Aaron and Miriam. So he departed from them. Miriam was afflicted with leprosy for seven days. Unlike man who looks at man, from the outside appearance, especially the skin color. God looks at the heart of man. *Moses' children were accepted as the same race as Moses, unlike today.*

Marrying someone from another race or culture can work out well if both parties are prepared for any negativity from others, and concentrate on building a strong relationship. In time, these negative outsiders will often end up regretting their negative comments as your relationship or marriage flourishes.

Some of you will make the conscious choice of staying single and will enjoy life without ever having a need to have a partner or kids. Others will enjoy the company of children by spending time with a favorite nephew, niece, or one of your friends' children. Avoid overindulging your friends or relative's child by overspending on clothes and other gadgets. A meal, walk, seeing a play, or spending time, or talking as you find out what is going on in their lives, are gifts that are irreplaceable.

Part III
Sexual Curiosity

Gender Challenged?

Psalms: 139:14
"I will praise thee; for I am fearfully and wonderfully
made: marvelous are thy works; and that my soul knoweth
right **well."**

Some teens become confused about their sexual identity before or during puberty. A boy believes he was supposed to be born a girl, and a girl believes she should be a boy. Some of these beliefs can be medically explained, others cannot. You might notice a boy displaying the characteristics of a girl, and a girl displaying the characteristics of a boy. It is important to avoid teasing these children as they work through this phase.

As you go through this perplexing stage, it will be hard for you to believe you are wonderfully made, but you are. Just look at your development from conception until now. Early, pastoral, and psychological counseling may be considered.

What About Teenage Sex with Consent?

1 Peter 5:8
"Be sober, be vigilant; because your adversary the devil, as a rowing lion, walketh about, seeking whom he may devour."

Puberty is often described as a difficult time, for some teenagers to control their raging hormones. "How can I keep mine in control?" You may ask. The longer you abstain from sex in any form, the easier it is to control them. Many have been disturbed after not experiencing the thrills they were made to believe they would enjoy. Not everyone gets pleasure on the first or second attempt. Trying to get that experience is what makes many keep trying. Abstention is still practiced today even though it is rarely talked about. Sex should be left for marriage then you can enjoy all its pleasures without the feeling of guilt and worry.

Guilt because you know it is wrong to give up your virginity this way.

Worry because even though you may or may not have used one of the many forms of birth control products on the market, none of them gives a one hundred percent guarantee against pregnancy, or a sexually transmitted disease. **Please note all forms of sexual activity carry the same health risk.**

All children do not listen to God's and their parents' advice to abstain and some do indulge in teen sex. Few practice safe sex on a consistent basis. Note that not all your classmates that are bragging about having sex are telling the truth, and if you dare to be different by not following the crowd, you can start a trend that will serve you well.

Some girls use abortion as a form of birth control believing that the unborn child is not a person. This is not true, as God says:

Jeremiah 1: 5:
"Before I formed thee in the belly I knew thee; and before thou comest forth out of the womb I sanctified thee, and I ordained thee a prophet unto the nations."

God knows each baby before he/she enters his mother's womb.
I do believe in choice because God gives us free choice, but given the facts, you will make better decisions. When a woman decides to terminate a pregnancy, without the correct intervention to save the life of the unborn baby, she will go to any length to do so. Before abortions were done legally, they were done illegally. The complications of an illegal abortion are far greater than those of a legal one, yet I have seen women lose their lives after having both procedures. Women that had an abortion, whether legal or illegal, may have difficulty forgiving themselves for their actions.

Matthew 11:28:
"Come all ye that are labor and heavy laden and I (Jesus Christ) will give you rest."

God is the only one that can stop the turmoil; just confess that you have done wrong and ask for His forgiveness. After you are forgiven, you do not have to carry that burden any more, so release it. You are now free; this is all it takes. Do not repeat this deed.

Sexual activity is a serious undertaking. For every deposit of semen that is deposited in your vagina, and vaginal secretions that enters your penis, a perilous residue may be left inside your body that may take years to manifest itself.

So each time you are tempted to have illicit sex, remember this hidden danger. Is taking the chance worth it?

If you are blessed to have a long term sexless relationship with your sweetheart in your youth, as you grow and see the sorrows that some of your peers that abused sex endure, please thank God for His grace for allowing you to know your teen sweetheart who did not even mention sex when you dated.

Yes, it is possible to date without sexual encounters. You set the rules. You do not *have to follow those that have many sexual encounters, making sex seem like you are going to a candy or toy store. Sex should be considered as a sacred act. Abuse may carry emotional, health and spiritual perils.*

Alternative Lifestyles

In Genesis 19:4-5:
"But before they lay down, the men of the city, even the men of Sodom, compassed the house round, both old and young, all the people from every quarter. And they call unto Lot, and said unto him. Where are the men which came into thee this night? Bring them out unto us, that we my know them."

This is the first account of homosexuality in the bible as the men of Sodom refused Lot's offer of his virgin daughters and demanded he give them the two men that had entered his house instead. God's anger was displayed as he destroyed Sodom because of it's immorality.

After going through the battle in their minds of which gender their bodies feel normal in, some boys/men choose the homosexual lifestyle. Homosexuality is found in almost all ethnicities and countries.

As a nurse, I have seen many young teens admitted to hospital for attempted suicide because they could not get their homosexual thoughts and longings to go away. Hence, I believe it is a spiritual struggle.

Some boys are molested by other males. Others have deliberately chosen this lifestyle, while some will tell you they believe it is how God made them. If this is so, would God keep all of your male and female organs functional, allowing you to have the ability to have children, knowing the turmoil your choice will bring to your children?

1 Corinthians 14:33
"God is not the author of confusion, but of peace, as one in all churches of the saints."

If you find yourself loving someone of the same sex more than you love anyone else it is possible to let him or her remain your best friend.

1 Samuel 20:17
"And Jonathan caused David to swear again, because he loved him: for he loved him as he loved his own soul."

Some choose to indulge in both homosexual and heterosexual relationships and are referred to as bisexuals.

When you hear the term "down low," what do you think it means? It took me a long time to find out what this slang meant. It refers to men who are married to women but are having secret homosexual relationships.

If you were to find out your spouse is involved in an alternative lifestyle, you will have to make the choice of what to do about you marriage. If you have difficulty, seek answers in the Word of God, pastoral or professional counseling.

Some people are born being part male and part female anatomically (this means they are born with male and female sex organs). Many times they may start out living as one gender, and as they age, they find out that anatomically and hormonally their shape and function is that of the opposite gender. This may be confusing and unbelievable to most. These individuals are referred to as being intersexed.

"Everybody needs somebody" and "there are not enough men in my city," is the excuse some females give for their lesbian relationships. In the Bible, it states that there will be seven women asking one man to carry his name:

Isaiah 4:1:
"And in that day seven women shall take hold of one man, saying, we will eat our own bread, and wear our own apparel: only let us be called by your name, to take away our reproach."

Nowhere in the Bible does it give you permission to take another female as a lover.

Job 19: 25-26:
"For I know that my redeemer liveth, and that he shall stand at the latter day upon the earth. And though after my skin worms shall destroy this body, yet in my flesh shall I see God."

You may have friends or family members who practice one of these lifestyles, and you may have difficulty handling your friendships. Continue to love them, pray for them, and lead them to the Word of God. We might not agree with His (God's) laws, but breaking any of them, including this one, is a sin.

John 3:17:
"For God sent not his son into the world to condemn the world, but that the world through him might be saved."

Ezekiel 33:11:
"Say unto them, As I live saith the Lord God, I have no pleasure in the death of the wicked; but that the wicked turn from his way and live: Turn ye, turn ye from your evil ways for why will ye die, O house of Israel?"

Proverbs 15:3:
" The eyes of the Lord is in every place beholding the evil and the good."

Here we see the Mercy of God. He gives us His Word (Jesus Christ) and Choice. He is happy when we choose Him.

I remember a friend, who is gay. When we met, there was an instant friendship. We ended up going to the theatre, shopping, and dining out. He wanted a friend at that time of his life, and I became his friend, simply a friend. I did not preach to him, neither did I go places that were exclusive to people that practice alternative lifestyles. It never came up. You can do fun things with friends or family members who practice alternative lifestyles without being tempted to cross over.

Part IV
Love

First Love

Teenagers often approach the person they have a crush on with their friends. If these feelings are not received well by the intended, the laughter and or jeers of their friends that might follow can often stop the rejected teen from ever approaching anyone of the opposite sex again. As you go through this stage be sensitive to each other's feelings. Try to approach the person alone, in case the feelings are not mutual, being turned down will not be so hard on your ego.

Most people remember their first love, which usually happens in their teens. To get that first love to feel the same emotions you feel is not always easy. Teenagers often seek their first love based on physical attractions or how smart or talented the person is. If you are short, you most likely will look for someone who is tall and vice versa. If you are very good at a particular sport or a gift in the arts, you may have many admirers to choose from. **Gladly, as we mature, we see that good looks and gifts are not always as important as what is inside a person's heart.** *As we go through life* many of us do not age looking like our teenage photographs. *Watch in awe as this unfolds. When you meet at your schools' reunion ten or twenty years from now, you'll observe the transformations of your peers, some natural, others cosmetic.* Many of you who are now classified as cute will no longer claim this title, and some that are average now will carry the titles of handsome or gorgeous. When I've met with some of my old classmates, the phrase we used is "God is good to us;" we are aging well. Doing our best to stay healthy and look our best do help. You can do the same so that when your class reunion rolls around, as you enter the room most of your classmates, will recognize you. You'll hear phrases like "you still look the same," or "you have not changed much." There will be no need to go on a drastic diet, do excessively strenuous exercises or have surgical procedures before the event.

As you find that special person, get to know each other well. If you watch some of the daytime TV drama programs and observe how often many characters change partners, you might think that it is impossible to find true love that last for years, but many still do.

Preparing for Marriage

Proverbs 18:22:
"Whoso findeth a wife findeth a good thing and obtaineth favor of the Lord."

As you consider marriage, if your husband finds you, I hope that many blessings are in store for you. You might say you found him but it is often the other way around. Many times, as we plan our wedding, we do not discuss some of the most important subjects that will help the longevity of our marriages. Here are some of the questions you should discuss with your potential spouse:

What is his or her religion? If you practice different religions, which one will you practice in marriage? How much time will you spend in church? Will you pray together? If you have children, which religion will you want them to practice? *It is important to note that although many people say they serve the living God, different religious conflict can still arise due to different doctrines, and this is sometimes hard to understand.*

If you are of a different culture or race, how are you going to blend both? Be aware a lot of negativity will come from outside sources. How will you deal with this? I have seen many men and women cry or become bitter at the negative comments or displays of others, because they were not well prepared for this behavior.

What does your partner think about marriage? What does he, or she, believe about the phrase 'till death us do part?'

How will you deal with your finances? Will you pool your money together or will you live like room mates, dividing every bill in half? *If you decide to do the latter, be aware that should one of you lose your job or become disabled, there is a possibility your marriage may fall apart or never be the same again. Some take this arrangement too far and are not willing to take on the finances of the sick, unemployed, or disabled spouse.*

How much of your money will you save, and who will take care of the finances? Take note that each partner should monitor how the money is being spent on a monthly basis. This is a good practice. Should the partner that takes care of the finances become incapacitated or dies, you will be prepared for whatever life brings your way.

How long will it take before you buy your first home, and how much of your income are you willing to spend on your home? Buying a home, depending on both incomes, may delay your wish to have a family, considering the high cost of real estate in most cities today. How long will you take to pay off your mortgage? If you live in a city with good public transportation, you may consider owning one family car and paying off your mortgage faster. If you decide to take 30 years to pay off your mortgage remember that house could end up costing you two to three times the initial price. Remember the days when everyone received a payment book for their mortgage, and paid off their mortgage, by making an extra payment any time they got extra money. In the case of illness, the family had a couple of months covered without worrying about losing their home. This is much better than saving money in an emergency fund at a low interest rate. Please note it does not matter how many extra payments you pay towards the principal of your house; if you cannot pay your current monthly payment, you can still lose your home to foreclosure. When you move into your first house, remember, it is not yours it's the bank's house. That is the reason why the bank forecloses the house you call yours if your payments are delinquent for a couple of months. If I could get something through to new home buyers it would be: Stop putting all of those expensive upgrades into the bank's house and see how soon you can acquire true ownership of the home. This will be a major accomplishment. After you own your home, you can do all your upgrades you desire.

Be wise; Proverbs 22:26-27: states:
"Be not thou one of them that strike hands, or of them that are sureties of debts. If thou hast nothing to pay, why should he take away thy bed from under thee."

We see many families that are victims of this, by the large numbers of the mortgage foreclosures presently on the market. *Using wisdom by paying off your mortgage as soon as possible cannot be stressed enough. It can save you thousands of dollars and help you avoid the likelihood of your family losing your home should illness strike or loss of income occurs.*

Keeping Intimacy in Marriage

Sex should be discussed, as it is an essential element in any marriage. Knowing your partner's expectations and desires can make your union go a lot smoother.

How many children will you have and what happens if there are no children? Can you have a happy marriage without children?

When you have children, will both parents continue to work? What about child care? If you choose to place your child in day care, how are you going to tackle the issue that may arise if your child is prone to infections and has to stay home until he or she is well?

It will be good to discuss what positive practices each of you can bring from your respective families to enhance your new family. Will you dare to talk about the negative practices of your family that you want to leave behind? Most people will not.

Who will be the cook in the family? If you both are accustomed to eating out, a few cooking lessons may be in order. Do not forget to share your favorite family recipes.

If they are any problems with the "in-laws," can they be resolved before you marry?

If you both have best friends, how are you going to fit these relationships into your married life? *Be aware that spending too much time alone with your partner's best friend of the opposite sex has ruined some marriages. He or she is your spouse's best friend, not yours.*

How does your partner feel about monogamy? Does your partner ever entertain thoughts of a threesome or wife swapping?

I do believe if these subjects are discussed, and couples are really honest with their answers, many marriages will not take place, leading to more happy families.

Keep the Spice in Your Marriage

Song of Solomon 4: 1 and 3

"Behold thou art fair, my love, behold, thou art fair; thou hast dove eyes within thy locks: thy hair is like a flock of goats that appear from Mount Gilead.

"Thy lips are like a thread of scarlet, and thy speech is comely: thy temples are like a piece of a pomegranate within thy locks."

The book of the Songs of Solomon shows us the sweet words of endearment Solomon used in courtship. *Most of us use similar words when we are dating but forget them soon after the wedding. Maybe we should record those lovely sentiments and replay them if we need to turn those sweet nothings into something to spice up our marriages.*

Some marriages become very boring soon after the wedding. Couples forget what brought them together, and do not realize that they have to keep the romance alive in order to maintain a healthy marriage.

If a marriage becomes boring, some turn to pornography, or an extramarital affair, believing it will bring spice into their marriage. Instead they create deception, worry or guilt, which is always followed by shame when exposed. Yet, many risk their marriage to indulge in these behaviors.

Pornography has a sneaky way of entering a couple's bed-

room. *It has two classifications, hard core or soft core. Hard core is bad and soft core is cool. So do not be deceived. It is an evil act in any form.* Once a person becomes addicted, "why do you think it is so hard to kick the habit?" God objected to the golden image His children made and worshiped, and I believe He feels the same way about those intimate objects made from plastic or crystal. Not all inventions of man are inspired by our Creator. If you are the innocent spouse, you must make sure you seek wise counsel. Wrong counsel will encourage you to be an active participant in your partner's negative behavior.

Avoid romance killers, such as: laying around in front of the television for hours with a remote control, becoming addicted to soap operas, lack of exercise, unhealthy eating and putting on a lot of weight in the wrong places, spending too much time talking to friends on the phone, not taking care of your hygiene and dressing sloppy when you go to bed.

Ignoring your spouse as you give all your attention to your favorite soap opera, ballgame or any television program has caused problems in many marriages. I remember a lady who visited our home. She had to remind me that soap operas are fictional. I introduced her to my husband, who came home for lunch, and I quickly turned my attention back to watching my favorite soap opera. I am glad to let you know I was able to get over my soap opera addiction shortly after her advice.

If you have someone at work who is spreading all the details of his or her toxic relationships. You should read;

1 Corinthians: 15:33:
"Be not deceived evil communication corrupts good manners."

The answer in keeping a marriage vibrant may be found by continuing to do what you loved doing when you were single. Was it dancing, going to the movies, taking long strolls together, a weekend away at a posh resort? Whatever you enjoyed doing together when you were dating include it in your schedule. If cost is a factor do it at least a couple of times a year. Seek new ways to spend fun time together.

The Wedding

A wedding can be a private ceremony, a beautiful affair for family and friends or an extravagant event. Some couples spend more time and money planning for their wedding than they take to plan for a healthy marriage. Yet an extravagant wedding does not mean the marriage will be a success. Many times the couple and their parents are left with bills that take many years to be repaid. *Repayment of this debt sometimes outlasts the marriage by many years.*

Set a realistic budget and stick to it. Do not burden your parents or take debt into your marriage. With a good wedding planner, you can have a beautiful wedding that fits within your budget.

I have attended some elegant weddings on a modest budget, which resulted in marriages that have outlasted some who have had extravagant weddings.

For those of you who can afford the extravagance, have a grand time, but spend just as much time preparing for a healthy marriage.

As you discus your wedding plans, take note of your intended spouse's attitude. Is he or she willing to consider your ideas? Or must everything be done his/her way? If this happens this sort behavior can dominate your marriage. Beware!

After the wedding, there comes the honeymoon. For the virgin wife, bleeding can occur when the hymen, which is a piece of flesh that covers the opening of the vagina, is broken. This might cause pain during sex for the bride and penal bruising for the groom. This may lead some new couples to complain that they did not find the "honey in the moon," while others said "it was like finding a good pair of gloves." Sometimes, it takes a while for the couple to get the gloves to fit correctly. (In Biblical times, if the hymen was broken before marriage, the bride and her parents were subject to public disgrace. (Today its' importance is often trivialized.)

Taking the name of your spouse is something that most women embrace. The women that keep their maiden names can be seen as rebels. I took my husbands name. Twenty years later I went to collect a copy of a birth certificate. When a name similar to my maiden name was called my heart started to race. Gradually it dawned on me that I was no longer called or known by my maiden name. After a few seconds, my heartbeat returned to normal. *So do not be so hard on women that may find it hard to give up their maiden names.*

Part V
Maturity

Becoming a Parent

Deciding to have children is a huge task and should be embraced by each parent. Each parent brings different values into the marriage. Knowing how to blend these values well can bring solace to your home.

Pregnancy may bring many challenges to a marriage. The expectant mother's body and emotions go through many changes. The father occasionally goes through an emotional phase. Some women are very beautiful during pregnancy, while others are not. Some trade in their beautiful figures for good. The father-to-be often feels left out as the mother's focus shifts from him to the pregnancy. Including your husband in the pregnancy as much as possible will make him feel relevant.

Good nutrition, exercise and a positive attitude are important to both mother and baby. Prenatal checkups, as ordered by your obstetrician, should be followed.

Today, most women are discharged from hospital after 48 hours of giving birth. I am glad this was not the practice when I had my babies, as I spent more than 48 hours with all of my children, and that is often needed. All women respond differently after giving birth, I know someone who can go to the movies three days after giving birth. This is unusual. It is a good idea to get a spouse or a relative to assist you for at least a week when you get home. This will allow you to rest and bond with your baby. Careful monitoring of baby and mother is very important, and any abnormality should be reported to your physician immediately. You should make sure your doctor does not dismiss your concerns without proper follow up.

If you can breast feed, I encourage you to do so. *Human milk is the best food for babies; "why else would God allow a woman's breast to create milk?" Yet I see many women who will not even consider breast-feeding and see the whole procedure as an unnatural act.* If breast-feeding is a challenge for you, let your nurse, a family member, or a friend who is experienced in the art to teach you how to conquer this technique. All babies do not acquire this natural instinct to breast feed before they are discharged from hospital. Therefore, first time mothers and mothers who have had long intervals between babies are often left alone to master this technique and often become frustrated and resort to bottle feeding instead.

If you choose to use bottle feeding, hold your baby close to your breast when feeding, making sure that the nipple is always full of milk and not air. Try not to prop up the bottle and let baby feed his or herself. Always burp your baby to release any wind or gas after each feed. Within months, your baby will be feeding him or herself.

Although we have so many toys and electrical gadgets to entertain and educate our children, do not forget about the human touch such as reading bedtime stories, singing, playing soothing music, creative play time, and going for walks.

Should you choose day care for your child, you should pick him or her at different times if possible. This will let you check out the activities, cleanliness and atmosphere of the school. "Would you like to be in this atmosphere for eight hours or more five days a week?" If the answer is no, you should consider looking for a new day care for your child.

Discipline is an area where many parents struggle today. *I often wonder what my father would think about "time out" being the recommended form of discipline.* I believe he would sit me down as we search the scriptures, as he waits patiently until I find and read:

Proverbs 23:13
"Withhold not correction from the child: for if thou beatest him with the rod he shall not die."

Yes, my father did use the rod, so did many other parents and teachers. I never saw a child who was seriously bruised or had to get medical treatment when a rod was used, and it did keep us in line. "Do I have flashbacks of being disciplined with a rod or switch?" I never do. Recently, one of my sisters reminded me that discipline did us good. It is not uncommon for a child to be beaten severely with injury, but as a youth, or a young nurse, I never saw that.

Although the law in your state may not let you use a rod to discipline your child, should your child break the law and is arrested, your child resisting arrest may be accompanied by physical "abuse" by law enforcement officers, which would cause you to be arrested if you had done the same thing to your child.

A practice I see too many parents comfortable with today, *is allowing their children to have sleepovers at a friend's house, without ever meeting or visiting the parents' home.* **Make sure you "*know*" and visit the parents at their home, before you give your child permission to sleepover.** *Parenting is always putting your children's safety first, this means saying "no" to your children at times.*

My first and only sleepover was at a friend's house that my Mum and Dad knew very well. I was supposed to spend the full weekend there. I was accustomed to having breakfast at an early hour at my home, but after a night of little sleep, the following day, it was almost midday and I was not offered anything to eat. I went outside to play, and saw a man from my village passing on his bicycle; I shouted and ran after him. He stopped, I asked him to tell my father to come for me, and he did. By the time my father came to collect me, I was still hungry. That was the last time I had a sleepover as a child.

When my last child was three months old, I took him to Bar-

bados to meet my family. I went to spend some time with a girl friend from school. I called my father and told him I was spending the night. When I returned to my father's house, I noticed my father was acting a little cold towards me. He soon called me aside for one of our little talks, and he let me know that the rules of his house had not changed, "sleepovers are not tolerated." I got the message and obeyed. Now that he is no longer alive, I spend many nights with the same girl friend when I am in Barbados. However unless I am out of town, as night draws near and my friends invite me to stay in their spare room, I think of my father and make my way home.

Young teens should be limited to the amount of time they spend talking to their friends on the telephone and computer. If you, the parent, do not know how to use the computer, get a pad of paper and pen, and let your child teach you. Taking notes will help you to retain the instructions. It is easy to learn if you approach it with the right attitude. Monitoring whom your young child is talking to on the computer is highly recommended, because there are many cases where children were hurt by the information they received, or from predators that surf the websites.

One of the joys a parent looks forward to is observing their children as they explore new and exciting experiences, but life also brings us sorrow. *Handling difficult situations effectively is when the true test of being a parent comes into play.*

Parents should be aware of their actions. Negative behavior is easily picked up by children and can become generational curses. These behaviors include things such as cursing, lying, cheating, gossiping, womanizing.

Psalms 34: 11:
"Come, ye children hearken unto me:
I will teach you the fear of the Lord."

Teaching children the fear of the Lord at an early age is the duty of every parent. Do not be perplexed by the fact that your child will not be able to talk about their faith in school; Jesus Christ warns us this will be common practice.

Luke 11:52:
"Woe unto you lawyers! For ye have taken away knowledge: ye entered not in yourselves: and them that were entering in ye hindered."

Barrenness

1 Samuel Chapter 1:4-6; 10-11; 20

"And when the time was that Elkanah offered, he gave to Peninnah his wife, and to all her sons and daughters, portions: But to Hannah he gave a worthy portion; for he loved Hannah: but the Lord had shut up her womb. And her adversary also provoked her sore, for to make her fret, because the Lord had shut up her womb.

"And she (Hannah) was in bitterness of soul, and prayed unto the Lord , and wept sore. And she vowed a vow and said O Lord of hosts, if thou wilt indeed look on the affliction of thine handmaid, and remember me, and not forget thine handmaid, but wilt give unto thine handmaid a man child, then will I give him unto the Lord all the days of his life, and they shall no razor come upon his head.

"Wherefore it came to pass. When the time was come about after Hannah had conceived she bare a son and called his name Samuel, saying because I have asked the Lord of him. Hannah kept her word and gave her son Samuel to the Lord."

1 Samuel 2:21:
" And the Lord visited Hannah, so that she conceived and bare three sons and two daughters. And the child Samuel grew before the Lord."

I was able to bring this story alive for the part owner of a store here in Florida. She had the same complaints as Hannah and her husband's former wife, who had children with her husband, took great pleasure in teasing her. I was blessed to witness a pastor whose prayers God had answered, and women, who had this problem, did conceive and had healthy babies. I asked her if she and her husband would meet with the pastor and she agreed. They met and within months, she became pregnant and had a healthy baby.

Recently I was in Barbados at a church convention when a visiting minister of God from Trinidad stated God is using him mightily in the area of infertility. When he asked those that were having problems in conceiving to come up to the front for prayer, the number of couples that are affected by infertility blew me away. Suddenly, it made sense as to why I had told my sister I noticed that not many Barbadian women are pregnant. I am glad to report that many couples became pregnant within months of that prayer.

Yes, God still opens up the wombs of women through prayer today.

There are doctors who specialize in the area of infertility, and some women do conceive after consultation and treatment. Using this method can be expensive but worth it for those who get positive results.

Yet, for you, pregnancy may remain a dream that will not be realized. Some women will become mothers through adoption, foster care, or caring for children as a live in nanny. This is God's divine plan. These women avoid the pain of childbirth while enjoying all the love, joys, and worry that motherhood brings.

Midlife

As you enter mid life you may be faced with different physical challenges. For a woman it is the menopause and for a man it can be andropause.

Menopause has two stages: Perimenopause and post-menopause. In the Perimenopause phase, your periods may become irregular or very heavy. Some natural remedies may bring you some relief. *A consultation with a naturopathic physician is important in ordering and monitoring the correct use of natural medicine and to alert patient of possible side effects.*

I remember a friend of mine who shared with me that he was admitted to the hospital many times because of episodes of a bleeding gastric ulcer. He was advised to take one cayenne capsules daily with a glass of cold water. He stated that the bleeding never recurred, hence eliminating the need for further hospitalizations. As I approached menopause, I used one capsule of cayenne daily during my periods. Do you know the phrase "there is nothing new under the sun?" Years later, I learned that some families have used cayenne as a tea for generations during menopause with positive results.

Some women with heavy irregular periods choose to have a hysterectomy. Remember that surgery carries risk, some of which can be fatal or more uncomfortable than a heavy period. Knowing at what age females on your maternal side went into their menopause can be helpful, as women from the same family seem to go into menopause around the same age. First consult with your physician to rule out any underlying medical problems. Then, decide if you can endure the discomfort of heavy periods if that maternal age group is not too far away. If a hysterectomy is your choice, be well informed before the procedure is done. Seek a second opinion from another physician if you have questions that are not fully answered. This will allow you to make an informed decision.

Post-menopause: your days of having a period are over. Some women complain of always feelings very hot for a short period (hot flashes), excessive perspiration and loss of sexual drive. This might be accompanied with excessive vaginal dryness, bone pain and weight gain. This is due to a change in the woman's hormonal balance. Your physician may prescribe medication to correct this. All women do not get positive results from these medications.

Resist the temptation to combine herbal and prescription medication, unless ordered and or monitored by your primary physician.

It should be noted that although many women in America go through many menopausal problems, the same does not apply to women from all countries; leaving one to believe it could be our diets and our lifestyles causing many of these problems.

For men who go through andropause, a sexual dysfunction such as impotence (which is the inability to obtain or maintain penal erection), they often find it a difficult issue to deal with. The cause can be mental or physical. Underlying issues such as prostate problems, diabetes, thyroid problems and high blood pressure may cause erectile problems. The side effect of some medication for these diseases may also cause erectile dysfunction.

Some men revert to the behavior of their youth such as dating someone much younger, going to activities mostly frequented by youth and updating their entire wardrobe and colognes. Sadly, these changes do not always improve their virility.

The following conditions can affect both sexes:

Short-term memory loss, such as misplacing objects like your keys, is a malady some experience during this phase. Retracing your steps, and making sure you consume foods that are high in antioxidants, that is fruits and vegetables that are rich in color, might improve this condition.

Impaired vision can also increase with the aging process. I believe that if we can get more seniors into printing and computer programming this problem will be not be as severe. I noticed impairment in my vision when I started to have difficulty reading fine print, and in time I started to use reading glasses. However, I became annoyed when I went to the supermarket and forgot my glasses, or I had to pick up my mail and not being able to sort through them without my glasses. I prayed that God would improve my vision. A friend of mine introduced me to a colorful nutritional drink. It tasted like an expensive juice, and I could not see any benefits. One day, as I was sorting the mail indoors, my sister, who was sitting at the dining table, said to me, "What are you doing?" "Sorting the mail," I replied. She asked me the same question three times and got the same reply. Then she said, "Where are your glasses?" "Thank God," I said. I soon found out that I could also read a newspaper outdoors; so now I do not have to go back to the car for my glasses when I go to the grocery store. Yes, I still need my glasses to read small print indoors, but I am thankful for the improvement.

Some people lose their teeth and wear dentures. If you are experiencing problems with chewing your vegetables blending or crushing your foods will help. Any natural fresh fruit or food that is slippery in nature may be of benefit; blended flaxseed can be sprinkled on salads and cereal. Do not forget to use healthy oils such as olive or cod liver as part of your diet. I watched a cook who prepared food for Pope Benedict use a very generous amount of olive oil. You will note that the Pope looks vey healthy. After writing my first book, I was questioned about the effectiveness of adding natural oils to your diet. Let me share this story with you. I bought into the fat free diet idea, so did my sister. Years ago, we were invited to lunch at an elderly couple's home. Soup was prepared for us and we were allowed to prepare our plates. We took pride in removing most of the fat from our servings. However, after observing that the couple was still in good health, into their late seventies, it dawned on us that this wise couple deserved the last laugh. Especially as I noticed signs of lack of lubrication in my body. *I often wonder, when did we start to see such an increase in hip and knee replacement and why?*

As couples go through these changes, some move to separate bedrooms and their relationship becomes that of a roommate or brother and sister, rather than husband and wife. Rarely do you find both partners comfortable with this living arrangement. *Couples should know that they can and should maintain intimacy such as hugging, kissing and cuddling, and eliminate the hurt that follows when one partner feels abandoned.* When I told my friend, who is approaching menopause and admitted to having some menopausal problems, to be aware of this trend, she gave such a hearty laugh of disbelief. However, for couples who are living this way, this is not a laughing matter. If God was able to revive Abraham at one hundred years and Sarah at ninety, He can also revive you. You may say moving to a separate bedroom has nothing to do with midlife issues; however, this is not a good way to spend your latter years. An appropriate intervention can bring you much joy and happiness.

If you are a couple that is enjoying this stage of your lives with favor, and the thought of separate bedrooms, is not an option, well done.

Empty Nest

Your children are grown and have moved out. You are excited about redecorating your home with all the upgrades you longed for; the high-end upgrades you know your children would not have appreciated and easily ruined. Be aware that many grown children return home with their own children, because of a negative event that has occurred in their lives. There go your upgrades. So many parents fail to teach their children how to appreciate these things and 'do not touch' can sound like a foreign phrase to some children. It is amazing how God prepares you for things to come. Once, a coworker who had car problems, asked me for a ride to work. She invited me in, as I was a little early. As I walked in, I gasped, "Wow"! "What happened?" I asked. "My daughter and her children moved in," she said. *You, too, might have to choose between giving your grandchildren shelter and enjoying your upgrades.*

Some couples decide to adopt a child or to become foster parents. If you have the energy this can be a good idea, and it can bring much love to you and the children in your care.

Others may adopt a pet; explore their own country or travel to other countries. Keeping busy as you continue to bring purpose to your life and the life of others should be your purpose. While some embrace this stage and would not trade it; others would do anything to recapture the days when their homes were filled with the laughter and activity of their youthful children.

Part VI
Lack of Love

Sleeping Around

This can be described as folly at a price, as many teens have been afflicted with a sexually transmitted disease (**STD**). When I was a teenager, there were two well known STDs, gonorrhea and syphilis. Both were treatable with a series of prescribed antibiotic drugs. Even though these STDs are still spread today, Herpes and AIDS are now in the spotlight; both of which have treatment available for their symptoms but no medical cure as of yet. There are also more new diseases, which we do not see in the news. Seek medical help if you believe you have contracted a STD and do not have sexual contact with anyone; this will help to prevent the spread of disease. Be aware, there are *some people who know they are infected and deliberately spread their diseases to others; this is a punishable crime in the United States of America.* Some teens might be too frightened to seek treatment for fear of parental involvement and will go to any length to keep this information a secret, leading them to go into a state of denial. Early intervention and treatment is important in combating these diseases.

Many of the things that give great pleasure also bring great sorrow. Having pleasure that is wholesome should be your goal in your youth, allowing you to arrive in adulthood with a healthy outlook.

Sexual Abuse

11 Samuel 13: 12-14; 19

"And she (Tamar) answered him, nay my brother, do not force me; for 'no 'such thing ought to be done in Israel. do not thou this folly.

"Howbeit he would not hearken unto her voice: but being stronger than she, he forced her and lay with her.

"And Tamar put ashes on her head, and rent her garments of divers' colors, that was on her, and laid her hands on her head, and went out crying."

*W*hen did the practice of displaying Tamar's grief at being sexually violated stop?

Sex is not discussed in most homes. It is often practiced behind closed doors. Thank God that today's parents are not telling their children that the stork brought the new baby. Television and the Internet have taken the myths out of what goes on in your parents' bedroom. Sex is normal, and it can be beautiful when it is performed in the way God intended it to be; that is between a husband and wife. Having sex any other way is accompanied by serious issues.

Sadly keeping sex a secret continues when most children are molested. There are some children that are abused by a parent, a stepparent, a sibling, an aunt, an uncle, a cousin, a teacher, a preacher, a boyfriend or girlfriend. Anytime someone forces you to have sex or invades your private space without your consent, it is sexual abuse. If this is happening to you, you do not have to keep it a secret. Telling a friend in most cases does nothing to stop the abuse, but allows you to share your pain. Do not blame yourself for this abusive behavior, believing you are responsible for this negative action. *As in many cases, the abuser might be highly regarded by your parents or members of society. You, the abused, have difficulty telling them that person they hold in such high regard has a dark side to him or her that has hurt you. "Who will believe me?" You may wonder.* Nipping the abuse in the bud will help protect you and others. Rarely does an abuser just abuse one person. *Do not even think of committing suicide or going insane, as some that are abused through incest do. You should confide in a trusted adult or teacher or report the abuse on the abuse hotline in your state. In America, sexual abuse is a crime punishable by the law and abusers are often monitored for years.*

Many that are abused as a child or teenager carry the scars for the rest of their lives; oftentimes affecting the relationship they will have with their future mate. Not all future mates will be aware that their partners' negative behavior during lovemaking has nothing to do with them. Although you may not be able to forget the abuse happened, you can see that it is not repeated, and you can grow up and enjoy a normal sexual relationship with your spouse taking full control of your life and your emotions. Professional pastoral or psychological counseling can help you to put the abuse behind you.

Sexual abuse, especially against women is a bigger problem in society than most believe. It has been so for generations. Put a group of older women in a room as teenagers talk openly about their abusers, and you will hear comments like "young people talk about everything today" or "child, get over it."

To you, the abuser, "Will you ask your victim for forgiveness for this evil act?" This can start the healing process for the abused and a change in your heart about repeating this behavior. Most abusers do not ask the abused for forgiveness, yet the abused

need to forgive the abuser to move on with his/her life. God says
we should forgive:

Matthew 6:12-13: states:
"And forgive us our debts, as we forgive our debtors. And
lead us not us not into temptation, but deliver us from
evil: For thine is the kingdom, and the power and the glory
for ever. Amen."

When you, the abused, forgive the abuser and/or the abused
asks for forgiveness; God can mend the abused heart and forgive
and change the abuser's heart.

Domestic Violence

This abuse can be verbal, non-verbal, emotional or physical.

As you discussed marriage and were setting up house together, you saw signs of abusive behavior in your spouse or partner, but you ignored that little voice that said "beware". You ignored the experts advice that says; "*It is often easier and less complicated to walk away at the first sign of this negative behavior.*" You willingly let him or her convince you that he or she was only joking or playing with you, when this negative behavior was first displayed.

Now, your abusive spouse or partner is taking control over what you say and do. You refuse to be controlled and a battle ensues. The abuser wins: you have the scars to prove it. Now you may even say that you never saw this behavior coming, but rarely is that true.

The negative behavior of the abuser is often learned and has been passed down through many generations, as the way of solving domestic disputes. Although this behavior can be changed with professional counseling and the renewing of the mind, many indulge in it for years, causing havoc in the lives of their victims. It is important to know that the abused cannot change the negative behavior of the abuser. It is up to the abusers to seek their own treatment.

I heard a minister, on a radio program, jokingly advising women to stop the divorces, endure the beatings of their husbands, and continue to pray to the Lord to change this destructive behavior. *Some Christian wives accept abuse, and have mental and physical ailments to prove it. Nowhere in the scriptures do I see it is all right to indulge in spousal abuse.* Too many countries and law enforcement officials do not take this abuse seriously. Some even think that women and men enjoy this as a form of love, as it is hard to fathom why the abused subjects his or herself to these repeated outbursts or violent attacks.

If you believe telling the abuser you are getting out of the marriage or relationship will cause you more harm, you should work out a safe way of escape. *Often with prayer and fasting, God will create an escape.* It is often impossible to get the abuser to seek psychological counseling, but you do have a choice and *there is help. In your local telephone book (in the blue governmental section in the United States) you can find the telephone number for the Domestic Violence Hotline. You can also check to see if there is a safe house for victims of domestic violence in your city.*

It is important to note that some of the abused are killed by their abusers when they decide to break up. **Therefore utmost caution must be taken when you decide to end these relationships.**

Do not let this negative behavior dictate the path your life will take, as some do, by going from one abusive partner to another or failing to ever trust or fall in love again. Knowing how you want to be loved and treated in a relationship is very important. Look for signs of negative traits that you will not tolerate in a relationship before setting up house. Move on; your life and sanity may depend on it.

Ending your Marriages

Many marriages end in separation or divorce, and this happens along all racial and religious lines. Trying to save a marriage before abuse, whether verbal, nonverbal, emotional or physical, gets out of control, should be a top priority for a couple. If this is not done, it often leads to the inability to save the marriage. Infidelity is often stated as a reason for the demise of a marriage. The guilty partner's refusal to work on saving the marriage, results in he or she seeking another partner who will make them happier. Often, this is only a temporary solution, as the incidence of divorce between couples of second marriages is even greater.

When we look at many of the men of God, in the Old Testament in the Bible, we see many of them had more than one wife. Today the injured wife may reciprocate by copying this negative behavior. The difference is that in biblical times all the wives knew one another and some even shared the same household, even though there were exhibitions of jealousy, the families were mostly intact. This was not the intention of God, as Jesus Christ pointed out, when he was tempted and asked if a man shall divorce his wife for every cause:

Matthew 19:4-6 and 8
"And he answered and said unto them. Have ye not read,
that He which made them at the beginning made them
male and female.

"And said, for this cause shall a man leave his mother and father, and shall cleave to his wife, and they twain shall become one flesh?

"Wherefore they are no longer twain but one flesh. What therefore God joined together; let no man put asunder.

"And he saith unto them, Moses because of the hardness of your hearts suffer you to put away your wives: but from the beginning this was not so: "

As we look at many children of divorce, we see that divorce was not a good choice for them. Parents may deny the fact that divorce affects the whole family, and the welfare of children is often not given adequate consideration. This does not mean that you should stay in an abusive marriage for your kids. If at all possible, you should work on rekindling the romance in your marriage for you and the kids, thereby, keeping the pledge you made to each other.

Often, when the divorce is finalized, one partner leaves the marriage and heads straight into another relationship. If you are the partner that is not in a relationship, it is not wise to rush into one just because you do not want to be alone. These relationships often cause you added pain because you are in them for the wrong reason. Allow your heart to heal from your broken marriage before entering another relationship.

A common complaint from the single divorcee, who had a healthy sexual relationship, is the sudden episodes of sexual desire that occurs without warning. If you believe God can take control of all emotions. *He will:*

Isaiah 26:3:
" Thou (God) shalt keep him in perfect peace, whose mind is stayed on Thee: because he trusteth in Thee."

Having a personal relationship with Jesus Christ can make

the transition easier as you go through the multiple emctions that often accompany a divorce. Having the support of family and friends is helpful. Unless couples seek counsel for the problem that caused their marriage to fail, there is a high possbility that the same problem can hurt their future relationships.

When you are ready to look for a new partner, if you have young children, make sure that the person is trustworthy and loves children. This is essential, as your new partner will become a part of your children's life.

A problem, you the divorcee, may encounter is dating and eventually marrying someone that is not as financially secure as you are. To protect your net worth and the welfare of your children from a previous marriage, you both might sign a prenuptial agreement. This can be a sound decision for some couples and is often entered in willingly by both partners. Yet, I have seen cases where the spouse, whose assets were less, walk away from the marriage, stating he or she does not feel trusted because they signed a prenuptial agreement. We live in a society where trust is not always present in a relationship. I remember a time when you got married and knew that your husband or wife would look after your children as their own, should you die, and the chance of a marriage ending in divorce was rare, thereby, eliminating or minimizing the need for such documents.

A negative trend, that some couples pursue, is constant court battles over child support and custody that can last for years after the divorce. *The money and time spent on these feuds will be better used for the welfare of the children: yet, the battle of retaliation of injured ex spouse continues to dominate our justice system. This negative behavior is not only harmful to the divorced couple but as long as it continues, it may affect any other relationship they are pursuing. How long are you going to carry on with this negative behavior? Let go and move on. The reason why you ended your marriage is so that you could start to enjoy life's hidden treasures.* Withholding child support is compounding the lack your children endure, and the emotional pain that occurs due to lack of your physical presence in the home. Show some love, for the welfare of your children.

If you are divorced and decide to setup a new family with children from a previous marriage, you'll have to decide how to combine both families, as your family becomes what is known as a blended family. It is not unusual to see one or more of the children, from either family, enter the new family with the intention of destroying it before it blends. Parents should be aware of this and nip the negative intent in the bud. If all parties of the blended family come into the union with the right intentions, the blended family can become a family to be admired.

If you are new to the dating scene after a long marriage, you must use caution. You will do well to read the advice given to teens about premarital sex and its hidden dangers. STDs do not respect age, profession, a pretty face or personalities. Many with positive attributes are infected with one or more of these diseases.

It is not unusual to see some divorcees make a decision never to marry again after going through a failed marriage, deciding to opt for a common law marriage instead. Some states have written laws to make such unions legal after a specified number of years. This may be good for the partners who give all of the support of a spouse but without the benefits.

Laying aside the hurt of a failed marriage proves to be impossible for many, so they go into new relationships expecting their new love to pay for all the past hurts of their failed marriage/marriages. This is a real turnoff. Many decide to remain single, rather than keep looking for someone who is capable of starting anew.

Few decide to let God become their husband as He said; serving Him as they do His work; enjoying the struggles and rewards it brings, as they keep in sweet communion with Him.

There is this old saying that "a *man likes to hunt.*" *That is why he finds it so hard to stay faithful in a relationship or marriage.* If you look at true hunters, they keep their catch. To me, man is like a modern day fisherman; he loves to show off his catch when it is

good but soon throws it back into the sea; hence, the trivializa-
tion of marriage.

Part VII
Death

Death of a Sibling, Best Friend or Class Mate

Matthew 5:4: states
"Blessed are they that mourn: for they shall be comforted."

The grief that often accompanies the loss of a child or a teenager can be devastating, and is compounded when the death is sudden or traumatic. I experienced such grief when my brother, who was two years older than I, died when he was nineteen years old due to an act of violence. Death is a natural event that can occur under unnatural circumstances, and although we know that we can die at any age, most children and their parents envision children will live to be adults and get to accomplish some of their dreams. *Parents of a deceased child often have a hard time coping with the death, and many voiced if given the choice, they would have swapped places with their deceased child.* Thankfully, most children grow up to be adults; hence this painful event is seldom repeated for most.

Pastoral and professional psychological counseling is good to help children and parents cope, yet it is wise to know that all of us should always be ready to meet our Redeemer (Jesus Christ) regardless of our age. I often hear people argue about when the end of the world will come. I never get involved in such argument. When you die that is the end of this world for you. This world will come to an end as the scriptures say. Making sure you live in a state of readiness is important.

Death of a Spouse

1Timothy 5:3-4:
"Honor widows that are widows indeed. But if any widows have children or nephews, let them learn to show piety at home, and to requite their parents: for that is good and acceptable before God."

The widow or widower is often very bewildered at the lost of his or her spouse. The deceased spouse is usually not the one that everyone, including the surviving spouse, expected to die first. Many spouses are not financially capable of taking care of funeral expenses; leaving them to seek help from family members and the church. Today, in some churches neither the pastor nor his assistants know their members. I find this baffling. As a nursing supervisor, if a patient was on a floor for more than a week, I knew that patient. Sometimes, I knew over one hundred patients at any given time. "Why do members feel lost in a church today?" As a pastor, do you or one of your assistants visit each member at their home at least once after they join your church? The world does a good job at running their organizations; what about you? Jesus Christ said that if a shepherd loses one of his sheep, he leaves all the others to go find that which is lost. I know a church family that relocated and they told me they were pleasantly surprised when the pastor, of a church they had visited, knocked at their door with a basket of bread and other goodies one afternoon. The couple appreciated this visit and joined that church. How many of your widows have not returned to your church simply because no one paid them a visit after the death of their spouse? What are you doing to educate your members to prepare for death should it happen prematurely?

Most funeral homes today will not take the body of the deceased until they are guaranteed payment. The bereaved spouse will do better by allowing the funeral director to take charge of the funeral arrangement therefore keeping cost within reasonable limits. This is not the time to go casket shopping. When I went through this, I did not look at caskets or pictures of caskets, the funeral director did a beautiful job. If your church is often burdened with requests for help with burial costs, you might consider starting a bereavement ministry.

Couples should make preparations so that the surviving spouse will be self-reliant especially if he or she will have to live alone. Losing a spouse should not be accompanied by losing everything you have worked so hard to achieve. The cost for this protection is often affordable if you buy it for protection purposes only. Some people will never own a life insurance policy, but setting aside savings or making alternative arrangements to cover your burial cost is essential. There is a misconception that the government will cover this expense. The last time I checked, Social Security paid less than $300 as a death benefit to those who qualify. With bad credit and no savings or insurance you might have difficulty securing a loan to bury your spouse.

Funerals are very expensive and it is your duty to make sure you take care of your spouse's expenses.

For children who have lost a parent, a good thing for you to do is call the surviving parent daily or to make sure someone else is doing so. Visit when possible just to show you care. Sometimes the surviving parent will not talk very much during your visit, but your presence will mean a lot. Pastoral visits during this initial phase will also be helpful.

In time, the grieving period will cease and the widow or widower will resume their activities of daily living, seeking what joys life has in store for them.

Part VIII
Challenges

Combating Illness

Knowing who to consult at the onset of illness may bring you wellness sooner. It is so easy to forget that God is the true healer. One evening, I was out of town and was about to go to church. As soon as I went outside, I started to itch all over my body. I was in a town that had no pharmacy in site. *My first reaction was, "I will not be able to go to church and will have to seek first aide to remedy this itching."* The evangelist that I was traveling with said, "What do you mean you are not going to church?" "Is church not for the sick?" *The nurse in me came up against the Word in him, and the Word won.* I went to church and before forty- eight hours without any medication the itching and rash had disappeared. Ever since then, at the first sign of any illness, I always consult God first.

Too many people claim diseases as their own. I do not know when this sort of thinking started. Talk to people with diabetes, high blood pressure, cancer or heart problems. They will say things like "my diabetes, my high blood pressure, my cancer," and the like. Being that these are destructive diseases that do your body harm, why do you claim them? You can eliminate them at the first sign of their invasion by acknowledging that good health is God's intention for you:

3 John 1:2:
"Beloved I wish above all things that thou mayest prosper and be in health even as thou soul prospereth."

If you have to take medication for these diseases; doing so as prescribed is important. Monitoring for effectiveness and side effects cannot be overemphasized. This is especially important when new medication is added to your regime. Remember, you must share information about any side effects with your doctor immediately. If they are extremely negative, stop taking the medication until you talk with or see your doctor.

Not all people have these diseases forever. With the Word, prayer, a change in diet, a well-balanced exercise regiment, and following doctor's orders, it is possible to eradicate many diseases.

What would you do if you had a wound on your leg, and you were told to put a bunch of figs on it in order to be healed? Or having leprosy you were directed to dip seven times in a dirty pool? What about hearing Jesus Christ the Great Healer was coming to town and all you had to do was to you touch the hem of His garment to be made whole. These were all miracles that occurred in the bible; so as we continue to make amazing discoveries in medicine, remember that God, who changes not, might use a simple remedy to cure your disease.

My son was involved in a car accident thirteen years ago. He was hospitalized for forty- eight hours. As soon as he got home he wanted to take a shower. I removed the bandage from his hand, and I was aghast at the condition of a laceration he had on the back of his hand. I had never seen a laceration that was so necrotic (dead tissue) in such a short time. I wondered what to do, as this was not an emergency, and taking him back to the hospital might have taken hours of waiting. A still voice said to me "*prepare* a piece of cactus (the type that some Antiguans and Mexicans eat, and Barbadians use to wash their hair) and apply it on his hand with a bandage." I did so and the next morning, when I removed the dressing, the wound was totally clean (pink). I applied vitamin E oil from a capsule for a couple of days, and the wound was completely healed within a week.

You might think this is foolish medicine, but it healed my son's hand. Maybe this was just a special cure for him. I am not sure, as I have never shared it with anyone to see if it will work for them.

You should always educate yourself before undergoing any invasive treatment, especially if it is not an emergency. Ask your medical practitioner to explain what the recommended treatment is in simple terms you can understand. He or she will likely comply. Information is also readily available on the Internet. If you are not computer literate, you can always get someone to do the research for you.

Today, many surgeries are done on an outpatient basis. This can give both the patient and their family a false sense of security. *Careful monitoring for twenty-four to forty-eight hours* after *discharging from hospital or clinic* is necessary, and it is wise to have a family member or friend to stay with you during this time. Remember, it was only a short time ago that many of these outpatient procedures required at least three days of hospitalization. *Any invasive treatment carries some risk.*

Disability

Disability affects people of all ages and races. *The treatment some employees receive when they become disabled can be described as heartless.* Employees that work with the same employer and in the same area for many years and suddenly become disabled. *If they did not make one or more personal friends on the job, in most cases they are forgotten, and treated as if they were never a part of the company; receiving no telephone calls, visits, get well cards or farewell party.* Even though they are severely disabled, they may have to hire an attorney to plead their case in order to be approved for the disability benefits they are entitled to. As this procedure can be stressful, some choose not to take this path, living in severe lack instead. *I did not know this problem was so prevalent, but as I age and see many of my friends and associates become victims of this practice, it has opened my eyes to this injustice.*

Many working people live from paycheck to pay check, not knowing when illness will strike. It is important to make sure that if you become disabled, you do not have to combine the stress of your ill health with the stress caused by the lack of finances, especially at the beginning of your illness. A lack in your finances, long term, is unavoidable for some, as many people cannot afford the premiums of an individual disability policy or do not qualify for these benefits.

If you feed on His word and believe in your heart as God states in:

Philippians: 4: 6-7:
"Be careful for nothing; but in every thing by prayer and supplication with thanksgiving let your requests be made known unto God. And the peace of God, which passeth all understanding, shall keep your hearts and minds through Christ Jesus."

Believe these Words and pretty *soon others will see a miracle in progress.*

It is also important to note that disability is more prone to happen in some professions than others. "Do you know the disability rating of your profession?" If not, please find out. This will alert you to employ all the safety measures that your job entails. Also to sign up for any employer sponsored short or long-term disability benefits. Be aware of when payment of both plans will start and how long they will last.

I do come across some people that appear disabled and still report for full time duty; only to end up being terminated for some cause and lose out on these benefits. Be wise. If you cannot do the job you were hired to perform effectively because of deterioration in your health, why report for duty?

There are children and young people who are disabled with different maladies. Their families can become stressed, especially if they are the primary care givers. It is wise for the primary care giver to take scheduled vacations to avoid burnout. Help from agencies who get funding from governmental agencies is available if the individual is preapproved. Working with a social worker who is knowledgeable about your case, can lead to finding the right avenues for assistance.

Today, so many of us do not want to intrude in the private lives of those around us. We believe the "if I do not tell you, do not ask me theory." Stand back and ask yourself, do you believe this theory should be used in all of life's situations? If you do not ask questions, how will you know if the person is well? This theory has left many in distress and in their homes alone for days. We will shout the most important things in our lives are God, family and our career. Yet our careers dominate most of our conversations with family and acquaintances. Due to the large number of broken marriages we would rather not hear how people families are doing. We miss out on the opportunity to give God blessings for those families that are intact, and to give comfort and prayer to those who are going through separation, divorce, illness, or mourning.

Retirement

Presently, I believe retirees fall into these six categories. See if you agree:

Group 1 "Making Dreams come true"

This group tends to approach retirement with such a zest for life. They may build their dream homes even if they are well into their eighties. Retirement is seen as a time to do all things they were too busy to do while they were working. They see it as a second chance to party, go to the theatre, dance, or to get that special sports car they always dreamed of. Some in this group still do all the vices that are done by the youth, such as excessive drinking and over indulgence in illicit sexual behavior.

 Is this the first time in history that people in their later years remained this active? No. Look at Joshua and many of the biblical heroes who lived more than one hundred years. This group reminds me of my youthful partying days when having fun was my main focus. How many in this group have fulfilled what God ordained them to be?

Group 2 "Returning to place of birth"

Retirees in this group cannot wait to return to their place of birth. Some return to the love of family and friends, while others become very lonely and live in isolation. This is often because many of their friends have either moved away, died, or react negatively to them, because they failed to keep in touch when they moved.

It is important that these retirees revisit their old hometowns for extended periods of time before the big move. Knowing how to make new friends by joining organizations that foster social activity can help to make the transition go smoother, allowing you to enjoy your retirement.

Group 3 "Awaiting the End"

These retirees are glad that they have made it into their seventies or older. They see it as a blessing and it is. They spend the balance of their life exerting as little energy as possible. They look forward to the end of this life and going to heaven. Sometimes, this group can spend days at home without daily contact with a family member or friend.

It is a good idea for a designated family member or a friend to make a phone call or to visit to these retirees every day just to make sure they are all right. Shut in ministry may be appropriate here. My question for this group is "why stop living life to its fullest so soon?" Considering many senior citizens are now living into their nineties, going to heaven takes a long time, and some are too eager to get there.

Group 4 "Keep on Working"

These retirees cannot afford to or choose not to retire. Either they need the additional income, or they believe keeping active will maintain their present level of functioning longer. They start a new career or they volunteer for some worthy cause.

Group 5 *"Old Age Mothering"*

These are the retirees who never get to enjoy retirement because they become full time mothers, a second time around. They take care of their grandchildren, or decide to take kids into foster care. Their children may be dead or are unable to care for their own children due to illness, imprisonment or drug addiction. Providing foster care may be done for additional income, as well as filling a need of giving a child temporary shelter and love. This group needs God's Strength and Mercy to endure. Any help that the church or the community can give is usually greatly appreciated.

Group 6 *"Living in Confinement"*

These are the retirees who because of poor heath, or poverty, spend the last years of their life bedbound or living in a nursing home, sometimes, never getting to go outside to feel the sunshine, or watch the sunset again. If you have a relative who is wheelchair bound, living in a nursing home and their medical condition allows it, see if you can get a doctor's permission to bring him or her home for Sunday lunch, a couple of times a year. This can be very therapeutic for the patient and good for the family.

Saving for retirement is a serious venture, but some people get so obsessed in making sure they are comfortable in retirement they sacrifice enjoying many of life's pleasures now. This is not wise; I have seen people who have done this die as soon as or before their retirement age. Although most of us will live to see retirement, there are no guarantees.

Although many employees are in charge of their own retirement planning, most do not understand their retirement plans.

While the cost of living in our country continues to skyrocket, many have lost some or most of the value of their retirement plans due to the instability of the international monetary markets. Worry and depression can set in as retirees agonize over their lack of finance, creating even more problems as their medical bills soar. Another thing that is causing much stress for seniors in my area, and is often discussed by retirees in the checkout line at local stores, is the escalating cost of homeowners insurance and property taxes. These costs have depleted many of their emergency funds in less than a year or two. You may ask me what I say when I hear the woes of these seniors. I say nothing. "My mind flashes to home owners whose insurance premium went from $153 to $532/ month; those who property taxes went from $6000 per year, to $10000/year; I think of you who have teenagers, who called me to see if I sell car insurance, because of the significant increase in your premium. It dawned on me that not only the senior citizens that are being affected, it is affecting everyone.

Part IX
Sunset

Sunset

I remember those wild flowers that swayed so gently in the breeze in the hills of Barbados. They did not bloom every year, and you could go years without seeing them, then they just reappeared. Life here on earth is something like that. We will disappear to reappear. We have to decide how we will return. Will it be a grand entrance or a sorrowful cry? Here are some scriptures that may help you make the right decision:

John 14:2-3:

"Jesus words are true when he said: In My Father's house are many mansions; if it were not so, I would have told you. I go to prepare a place for you.

"And if I go and prepare a place for you, I will come again, and receive you unto Myself; that where I am, there ye shall be also."

Acts 16:31:
"And they said, Believe on the Lord Jesus Christ, and thou shalt be saved, and thy house."

11 Timothy 2:12:
"If we suffer, we shall also reign with Him: if we deny Him, He will also deny us."

11 Corinthians 5:7:
"For we walk by faith, not by sight."

Hebrew 11:6:
"But without faith it is impossible to please Him (God): for he that cometh to God must believe that He is, and that He is a rewarder of them that diligently seek Him."

How much thought do you give to life, the second time around? Are you following Christ's command to go into the world (the world, to you, may be anyone you come in contact with) and tell others that Christ paid the price for their sins and they must repent to be saved?

Or are you consumed by riches and the cares of this world? If your riches consume you, be aware that many that follow this path die and leave their wealth behind and those that inherit it, may squander it.

1Timothy 6:17:
"Charge them that are rich in this world, that thou be not high minded, nor trust in uncertain riches, but in the Living God who giveth us richly all things to enjoy."

Have you considered sharing your wealth with the needy? You do not have to tell the world about your good deeds, receive your reward openly from God instead.

Matthew 11: 28-30:
"Jesus said, Come unto me, all ye that labor and are heavy laden, and I will give you rest.

"Take my yoke upon you and learn of me: for I am meek and lowly in heart: and ye shall find rest unto your souls.

"For my yoke is easy, and my burden is light."

Ask Jesus to come into your life and forgive your sins today: He will. It is that simple.

The choice is yours to be with God, who is Light or to be with the Devil, which is darkness. Who do you choose today?

At puberty the thought of your life having to end seemed so far away. Anyone that prepares to go into the sunset (die) will tell you that this journey called life is just a blink. Our next life lasts for eternity, and eternity has no end.

www.ingramcontent.com/pod-product-compliance
Lightning Source LLC
Chambersburg PA
CBHW070834310526
45788CB00017B/709